HEALTHY SMILE, HEALTHIER LIFE

*The health signs your dentist can
see that your doctor didn't tell you about!*

Kevin H. Norige, D.M.D., F.I.C.D

Foreword

My father died of cardiac disease in 1985. Now, I know that my father went to the dentist all the time and I know he had crowns and bridges and all manner of dental work. Unfortunately, I'm absolutely positive he didn't have any gum treatment done because it simply wasn't done back then. More recently, scientific studies are proving there is an intimate relationship between the mouth and the heart (as well as the rest of the body). If only we had known back then...

I want to help as many people as possible to become more knowledgeable, to become healthier. To do that I can relay the information, but the patient needs to take responsibility, to be answerable for his own health. I hope that by sharing information through this book in an easy to understand fashion many people will take charge of their health care, and stop relying on sick care.

About the Author

Kevin H. Norige, D.M.D., F.I.C.D. is a prominent dentist and lecturer focused on oral health as part of the whole body system. Dr. Norige is Chairman of the Connecticut State Dental Association Annual Scientific Session, a Fellow of the International College of Dentists, Member of the exclusive Horace Wells Club, and maintains membership in the American Dental Association, the Hartford Dental Society, and the American Academy of Oral Systemic Health. Dr. Norige has been a preceptor at the University of Connecticut School of Dental Medicine, an adjunct professor at St. Joseph's College, and Co-Chairman of the Connecticut State Dental Association's Pregnancy Clinic at the annual Mission of Mercy.

Dr. Norige has provided dental care to patients in four countries in North and Central America, as well as patients from Sweden, Uruguay, Venezuela, and China. Dr. Norige has experience treating people from a wide range of backgrounds: doctors, lawyers, bus drivers, retirees, and professional athletes.

Dr. Norige has been seen on "Better Connecticut" and "Eyewitness News" on WFSB Channel 3, heard on "Between Rounds" on WTIC 1080, and in an exclusive interview on eHealth Radio. Dr. Norige has had multiple articles published in "Natural Nutmeg" magazine. As a speaker, Dr. Norige has appeared at the Rotary Club, the Chamber of Commerce, the Boy Scouts of America, privately owned dental practices, and local schools.

Dr. Norige's office is located in South Windsor, Connecticut, and he enjoys his time off on the Connecticut shore with his wife Donna. Dr. Norige is a voracious reader that enjoys nature, hiking, and biking. Dr. & Mrs. Norige enjoy time with their son's and daughter's families, and most especially their four grandchildren.

Dr. Norige is available for a limited number of speaking engagements each year. For more information, visit www.Kevin-Norige.com.

To contact Dr. Norige's dental practice regarding dental care, please visit www.SouthWindsorSmiles.com.

CONTENTS

"Listen Up, Doc."

One young lady came in to see us and found she needed to have some restorative work on a few teeth. She then expressed her biggest concern, "It takes me a long time to get numb." Somewhere in her past experience with other dentists she found herself in a painful position when anesthesia hadn't set in completely prior to the start of dental work. I can certainly understand her apprehension to have dental work done after that experience, so we listened.

On the day of her appointment we got her in an hour earlier than her appointment time, just to get her numb. It worked! She was so happy it didn't hurt and we didn't treat before she was numb that she actually told us in disbelief how proud she was that "we listened!".

How well is your doctor or dentist really listening to you?

Instead of invoking the famous cartoon quote "What's up, Doc?", and opening the door for the practitioner to talk, you might want to say "Listen up, Doc.", to make sure that your practitioner is listening to you.

Have you ever been to see a doctor or dentist and felt like he or she wasn't listening to you?

Did it seem that they were waiting for you to finish speaking so they could tell you what they think... without hearing or understanding your true concerns?

Unfortunately this is common, and everyone does it from time to time. We observe and fill in the blanks before we get all the data (sometimes even interrupting to try and finish other's sentences).

It's dangerous when physicians fall into this very human trap. Diagnosing and recommending treatment before "listening" and gathering all of the data can have disastrous consequences.

I saw a patient recently who had stents placed a few months prior to our visit. His blood pressure reading at our visit was abnormally high, and I informed him that we would not complete the treatment at that time due to the high blood pressure reading. It was then that he told me he had simply forgotten to take his blood pressure medication that morning.

For some physicians that would have been the end of the interaction. For others, the conversation would continue because it was quite clear that this patient didn't understand how his blood pressure medication worked, and did not fully feel the weight of the consequences of not taking the medication as prescribed (blood pressure medication is not like taking aspirin and feeling better twenty minutes later).

This example demonstrates that the opposite line of communication must also exist. The physician has to make sure that the patient understands what is recommended, and it is the patient's responsibility to keep asking questions until complete clarity on the situation is reached.

Quite reasonably, a physician taking the time to learn about the person as more than a symptomatic body part feels like real, genuine care.

I believe this is why eastern medicines are gaining popularity in our culture, because there is more of an effort to find out more of what's going with the person overall, rather than just looking at just one symptom. Any one sign or symptom usually doesn't tell the whole story.

What is Complete Health Dentistry?

The mouth is a window to the rest of the body. If something is going off the rails in the mouth, what else in the body is negatively affected? Conversely, if we correct an issue in the mouth, what are the positive effects that will be found elsewhere in the body? Most physicians (and more dentists than you'd think) haven't even considered this possibility.

We routinely offer to take BP at office visits, and we get plenty of people who don't want to have their BP taken. I understand. They're afraid, because once they know, they have to deal with it.

Recently, a male patient in his late fifties had a high blood pressure reading at our office. I advised him to get it checked by his physician, which he did.

And the first thing his physician said was, "Why is your dentist taking a blood pressure reading on you?" And then... she proceeds to take his blood pressure again — *only to put him on blood pressure medication that day!*

She never would have known, had his dentist not taken his blood pressure, at least not until his next physical, or until he had a stroke as his terminal event.

This sort of short-sighted thinking is what complete health dentistry is looking to change. There is no reason that highly trained medical professionals can't recognize health concerns that are better addressed by dentists, and the opposite is also true.

Most dentists are only focused on looking at teeth as teeth, and gums as gums. They have forgotten to put the mouth and the body together as an integrated whole, meaning that the teeth, gums, tongue, cheeks, lips, throat, and other associated organs, are in fact pieces of the whole body puzzle. Evaluating the information from each piece of the puzzle can give us the whole picture, and correcting one issue can actually change the whole picture. That is what complete health dentistry is really all about.

It should be the job of everyone in the dental and medical fields to help people by evaluating signs and symptoms of a condition or dysfunction to determine its root cause, and then to address that cause rather than just the symptoms. One example where dentists can help is when we find periodontal disease ("gum disease"). We know the serious consequences of bacteria of the mouth relative to heart disease, and we should be talking with the patient and their primary care physician about these dangerous connections. Dentists can see signs of many whole body, or systemic, issues and relay that information to the patient's primary care physician while concurrently working to eradicate infection and disease in the mouth. This book addresses some of these life-threatening systemic issues as seen from the point of view of a dentist.

The Traditional View of Periodontal Disease

Gum disease is a misnomer.

When a person has "gum disease" the gums are indeed diseased, but this is merely a description and a name of an anatomically localized group of signs and symptoms. A wide array of treatments and therapies exists with varying degrees of success in achieving optimal health because of this symptomatic description and name. Better outcomes would be delivered if a focus on treating the root cause(s) of this disease, were involved and applied.

Gum disease (technically the spectrum of periodontal diseases including gingivitis and periodontitis) is the combination of:

1. the localized and overt manifestation of the systemic (whole body) condition known as inflammation and;
2. an aberrant oral ecological balance (more bad bugs than good bugs).

Before the modern era, "pyorrhea" was the term used to describe the collection of observations connected with "bad gums". The term pyorrhea comes from the Greek, literally meaning "pus flowing condition". This collection of observations included stinky breath, swollen and red gums, loose teeth, and blood and pus coming from between the teeth and gums. The usual outcome of this condition was the loss of teeth and the need for either partial or complete dentures. And as this condition always seemed to be associated with aging, it was felt to be an inevitable consequence of the aging process.

Currently the dental profession recognizes eight major different categories of "gum disease". And yet, even with all manner of treatment modalities extending from lasers, surgeries, scaling and root planing, antibiotics, disinfecting solutions, and trays to the mundane and historical brushing, flossing, tooth picking, water picking, and various toothpastes, "gum disease" continues to be the most prevalent chronic disease known to mankind.

The artificial separation of the oral cavity from the rest of the body and the treatment of diseases that show up there leads to management and treatment of those diseases that is compartmentalized, symptom based, and mechanistic rather than directed at the root cause of the problem. The underlying problem is that we're looking at this condition through the wrong paradigm. We're looking at these conditions as "gum disease" rather than as the local reaction to systemic disease combined with a biological bacterial imbalance. Because of that view, we're not as successful as we could be in managing these conditions.

When we view periodontal disease beyond merely the response of our gums to pathogenic microorganisms, we can develop better and more complete treatment modalities to solve that problem for that individual. For example, brushing and flossing are important, but those efforts are limited in their effectiveness because we are primarily treating symptoms, rather than addressing the larger issue of that particlular individual's whole body response to the wide array of inflammatory system actions and ecological imbalances. What might happen if we treat the whole body while also providing care for the afflicted areas in the mouth?

The Double-Edged Sword

"Your mouth is your foundation for health, and the way you treat it is the exact way that your body will treat you back."

(Dr. Steven Lin, <u>The Dental Diet</u>)

Inflammation is the double edged sword in health and wellness.

So, what is inflammation? Inflammation is the term used to describe the body's usually protective responses to any kind of particle (living or non-living), energy (light, heat, electromagnetic) or trauma that impacts the individual. The four classic signs of inflammation are: "rubor" (redness, due to increased blood flow), "tubor" (swelling), "calor" (increased heat or temperature), and "dolor" (pain). Another characteristic of inflammation is that it is not specific to a particular type of insult, but has very generalized effects on tissues and organs not involved directly with the insult, that is to say, systemic effects.

There are two major types of inflammation: acute (the body's response to the perceived insult seems appropriate and in limited duration proportionate to the degree of problem presented) and chronic (the body's response persists beyond the need to handle the insult and the inflammation itself becomes a new and persistent problem). As the response to an assault on our bodies' functional integrity, acute inflammation is necessary to life and living. But as an inappropriate prolonged action, chronic inflammation can be disabling or even life threatening.

Chronic inflammation spreads easily throughout the body because everything in the body is affected by and connected with the vascular system. Chronic inflammation occurs when acute inflammation continues for too long — the body forgets what turned it on in the first place, so it just keeps running, causing a sort of inflammatory overflow. When an overflow occurs the inflammatory response will first affect the circulatory, or vascular system, before spilling into the next most susceptible body system and ultimately to other parts of the body.

If the vasculature gets fouled up, you run a high risk of multiple dangerous conditions to your health. For example, there are chemicals that our body's fight cells release that make bacteria more tasty to the bacteria-fighting cells. These chemicals are called immuno-globulins. Imunnoglobulins attach themselves to bacteria or viruses or whatever is the noxious intruder and it makes them more appetizing to our phagocytes — our cells that eat and destroy these threats in our body.

The problem is that immunoglobulins can get overzealous and start thinking healthy cells are bad. When this happens the immunoglobulins attach themselves to healthy body cells prompting an "attack" by our body's defense system. This is an easy way to understand auto-immune disease, and the potentially huge negative effect of inflammation on our health.

Inflammatory Response and Diet

*"In reality, what's good for the mouth is good for the rest of the body...
(a healthy diet) helps to prevent disease not only in the mouth, but in your bones, gut,
immune system, and brain as well."*

(Dr. Steven Lin, <u>The Dental Diet</u>)

When we get too much sunlight we get sunburn. The body is telling us "get out of the sun!" And sunburn can be painful, so what do we do? We use anti-inflammatories and cool the affected area of the body down again.

The same thing happens on the inside of the body. Arteries get inflamed when we feed the the body too much of certain foods. For instance, if we give it too many refined carbohydrates. Refined carbohydrates taste good, they look good, they're fun to eat, and they give us an immediate high and boost of energy.

But what happens when we crash? The body has to recalibrate, reacclimate, readjust. But we usually don't give the body time to do that because now we give the body another dose of refined carbohydrate. We become addicted to this outside stress called "food", instead of saying "How hungry am I really right now?" "Do I really need to eat, or only want to satisfy my craving?"

Are You Fueling Inflammation and Illness?

60% of foods eaten in the Standard American Diet promote chronic inflammation.

The major culprits are:

- Refined sugar

- Refined grains

- Grain flour products

- Refined oils (including: corn, sunflower seed, safflower seed, cotton seed, peanut, soybean)

(David R. Seaman, DC, MS, <u>The DeFlame Diet</u>)

Unfortunately the modern standard American Diet is a very sad diet and feeds our food addiction or craving. What happens when we eat a diet high in refined carbohydrates is that we don't get enough fiber. All the fiber has been taken out when we refine whole foods into refined foods. The whiter the product is, the worse it is for you when it comes to breads and sugars. (Limiting the amount of whole wheat bread is also good for you because of other additives and preservatives.) This is because they are all processed foods that have essentially eliminated the fiber that is good for you, leaving nothing but simple carbohydrates (simple sugars, which are quickly broken down by our body requiring us to refuel rapidly). Unfortunately if that food energy isn't used right away it is stored for later, and this leads to the depositng of abdominal fat which is so very bad for us.

We know that diabetes is a scourge and is going up at an astronomic rate. Metabolic syndrome, which includes high blood sugar, is caused mostly by not eating properly. Metabolic syndrome is a catch phrase for a multitude of signs and symptoms including obesity, high blood pressure, and insulin resistance — which causes diabetes. A syndrome is not a disease by itself. It is a collection of diseases, potential diseases, and symptoms that together yield a particular result for the practitioner to look at to find the root cause(s) and appropriate treatments.

So where does fiber come from? Fiber is the pulpy, stringy stuff in celery, or an orange, etc., and that fiber holds things together. What it does is provide a food source and a place for the good bacteria to live and proliferate. Fremented foods are another good source of fiber for those good bacteria to live on, plus the added benefit of containing certain strains of good bacteria.

We have to get back to the concept that food is medicine.

The correct food, real food, is not in processed food. Raw fruits and vegetables are the best food we can consume for our health. We think there is a lot of sugar in fruit, and there is, but there is also a lot of fiber — and the sugars in fruits and vegetables are complex carbohydrates so they process more slowly than simple sugars. As an aside, cooking may not be the healthiest way to prepare our food. The chewing of raw fruits and vegetables required for digestion is also really important for the appropriate development of the bones of the skull and the facial muscles so that we get proper alignment of the teeth, and it also helps fight cavities and inflammatory gum disease, as well as provides proper development of the nasal cavity.

We are living in the era of a food processing health nightmare. The USDA had their food pyramid and it was eat lots of carbs, less meat. It became inculcated in dietary process. More recently we've learned we need to eat meat — and especially *grass fed meat* because it has other important benefits than protein and fat (for more on grass fed beef, see page 53). (Even cattle lacking their natural diet get these diseases — and then they have added antibiotics and growth hormones to correct for these dietary deficiencies. And then those pharmaceuticals are transmitted into the population that eats the meat, or drinks the milk.)

Studies have shown that Asians who have emigrated to the United States, now using rice that has been stripped of its fibrous hull, have begun to get the same diseases that Americans alone were getting as a result of a heavy processed foods diet. It's sort of a nod to Weston Price, a Canadian dentist in the early 1900's, whose research demonstrated that if people stayed within their native diets they were less prone to dental disease like cavities, inflammatory gum disease, and crowded teeth.

He was on to something. Our diets greatly affect our overall health and wellness, with a myriad of diseases able to be prevented by maintaining a healthy diet, yes, food is medicine.

Dietary Effects on Breathing

Research strongly indicates that the American diet over the last 70 years has caused an amazing increase in people having to breathe through their mouths, and not coincidentally an increase in the number of people suffering from sleep disordered breathing.

If you go back before World War II, you had to cut your meat, eat your potato, eat your vegetable, chew and then swallow. Chewing seems to force the muscles to force the jaws to work where they're supposed to be, so it keeps the jaw and the facial form aligned normally.

With the advent of mass produced, manufactured, homogenized foods (hamburgers, chicken nuggets, soft breads, processed meats, precooked soft and mushy foods) the jaws don't have to work quite as hard. Because you don't have to chew hard, you aren't developing the musculature that will force the jaws to work where they are supposed to be—causing a narrowing of the jaw and a vaulting of the palate (which in turn compromises the nasal airway).

Different cultures have different facial forms, but when you look at primitive cultures that eat raw foods most of the time, they don't have these issues, like obstructive sleep apnea. You'll see popular diets come and go, but the fact is, the more raw food, especially fruits, vegetables, seeds, and nuts that are in your diet the healthier you will be.

Breathing and Oxygenation

*"We've all been told that diet, exercise, and a good night's sleep
are the keys to handling life's stressors. But being able to take
a deep breath is equally important."*

(Gelb and Hindin, <u>GASP</u>)

The body needs oxygen — it's our primary nutrient. You cannot live without oxygen for more than 3 minutes. You can live without water for around three days. You can live without food for around thirty days. But oxygen? You've got to have it. And if the body's vascular (or circulatory) system gets clogged up, the oxygen can't get to where it is needed. For example, if you whack your hand it starts to swell and that swelling slows down the circulation. Next, the area gets black and blue, and yes that is blood getting out to where it is not supposed to be, but it is also a lack of oxygen in those body tissues. The bluer the area, the less oxygen is present. And how do we obtain more oxygen? We breathe.

Breathing correctly means breathing through the nose, not through the mouth.

Inside the nasal passageway there are horizontal bones called turbinates that warm and moisten the air entering the body. If you breathe through your mouth you can get a lot of cold dry air going into the lungs and that can actually hurt your lungs. Turbinates also have another function, they grow lots of tiny hairs to filter the air and take a large portion of the dust, pollen, and other particles out of the air before the air can enter your lungs.

Another reason that nasal breathing is so important is that nitric oxide gets formed In the mucous lining of the nasal cavity. A lot of compounds containing nitrogen and oxygen together tend to dilate blood vessels. Compounds like nitro-glycerin, nitric oxide and nitrous oxide, for example. And when we dilate, or open, the blood vessel it allows for blood to flow more freely. What happens then is the necessary oxygen can be transported through the bloodstream to the peripheral areas of the body (like fingers and toes), and it allows the body to get rid of the carbon dioxide and all cellular waste.

When we improve blood vessel flow we're going to improve oxygenation of the tissues and when we improve oxygenation of the tissues they function properly (and painlessly minus other extenuating circumstances). Pain and inflammatory response are increased when oxygen and blood flow are diminished. For example an eschemia, which is why we get pain in the heart during a heart attack, happens because those blood vessels close down and the muscle of the heart is working hard without enough oxygen and the heart muscle gets sore.

This may sound unbelieveable, but we really need to learn to breathe through our noses properly. Frequently pollutants and allergens compromise nasal breathing, even in somebody who has anatomically normal pathways. When your nasal pathway gets swollen due to the pollutants and allergens it can't do its job. It can't warm the air, filter the air, moisten the air, or produce nitric oxide, because you respond by breathing through the mouth.

Most of the time mouth breathing causes us to breathe too much. We become hyperoxygenated which isn't ideal. The mouth opens and sucks in too much air, so our lungs don't get to exchange carbon dioxide for oxygen. Too much or too little oxygen (or anything else) is bad.

Earlier I made reference to a person having anatomically normal pathways in regards to proper breathing. What I mean basically is that there is an appropriate airway opening that allows for sufficient airflow through the nasal cavity. This may be a surprise, but if you expand the palate (the roof of the mouth), you create an open passageway for better nasal breathing.

The palate should be horizontal. But, if it is not allowed to develop that way, it tends to become peaked, very high, vaulted and narrow. When you have a peaked palate the force put onto it begins to concentrate, and the bones begin to develop tori. Tori are bony protuberances in the palate that compromise the space where the tongue should be even more. When this space is reduced there is no room for the tongue, so it has to go down and back, blocking the back of the airway. As the palate becomes more pointed and less rounded, that reduction in side-to-side space in the nasal cavity causes the turbinates to get smooshed together and tilted upward, reducing their effectiveness.

The same thing happens with the mandible (the lower jaw). The mandible is supposed to be "U" shaped, creating a broad visible smile surface across your front teeth (the bottom of the "U" being the front teeth). As the lower jaw and palate become more pointed and less rounded they form more of a "V' shape, creating a narrow visible smile surface (the bottom of the "V" being the front teeth). When the palate is narrow, the mandible will be narrow as well, so you get more tori, and the tongue can't lie on the floor of the mouth like it ideally should.

By intentionally broadening the palate through orthotropics (commonly referred to under the umbrella term of orthodontics) we can create space and parallel the turbinates. With that adjustment you'll get corrected air flow through the nasal cavity. For children, whose skulls are still growing and developing (up to the approximate age of twelve years), a healthy diet of not-overly processed foods can help broaden the mandible and palate naturally creating space in the nasal cavity.

Signs of Airway Obstruction in Kids

- Mouth breathing

- Open or slack-jawed posture

- Snoring or noisy sleep

- Night terrors

- Bed-wetting

- Chronic runny nose

- Chronic ear infections

- Dark circles under eyes

- Tossing, turning, thrashing and restless sleep

- Messy sheets and blankets

- Nail-biting

- Crooked teeth

- Frequent earaches

- Falling asleep in school

- Awakening feeling unrefreshed

(Gelb and Hindin, <u>GASP</u>)

Sleep and Oxygenation

"Sleeping and breathing are things that we all take for granted... and when we don't sleep well, we'll be wondering how we can sleep better the next day. No one ever realizes that they did not sleep well because the were not breathing well."

(Steven Y. Park, M.D., <u>Sleep, Interrupted</u>)

Have you ever looked under the eyes of a person, and they have those dark circles under the eyes? It means they are not getting oxygenated. When does that oxygenation occur? At night, in the non-REM deep sleep — the deepest level of sleep. And you don't need a lot of it, but you do need enough of it otherwise you age, you get worn out, you get tired.

We had a patient in just the other day, and I could see wear on his teeth, and I said, "Do you grind your teeth at night?" (Grinding is a constant rubbing back and forth of the teeth. This is going to wear down your teeth, just like rubbing two rocks together will wear down the rocks.)

He said "Yeah, I do."

I said, "Let me ask you a second question... have you ever been told you snore?"

He sat back and his eyes popped open and he said "Yeah, how did you know that?"

How did I know that? And why would I be concerned about that?

Well sometimes the grinding we see is the body's response to try and open the airway up with musculature moving the jaw forward, and then relaxing in a cycle. Why? Because you aren't getting enough oxygen, and the body is trying to survive. Yes, to answer your question, other things like anxiety can contribute to this activity, but during sleep it is primarily a defense mechanism for your body.

Grinding is just one sign that dentists can see that might signal a sleep breathing disorder. Snoring is another. By recognizing these signs I can understand that your breathing may be disordered, and now I can refer you to your physician and have you demand a sleep test. Sleep test results in the right range allow your dentist to help you with an oral device (yes, there are alternatives to C-PAP machines that work for some people) that will not only prevent you from grinding your teeth, but also lengthen your life because you can breathe better during sleep. (A side bonus: you won't feel tired "for no reason" in the middle of the day anymore.)

Why is a dentist concerned about sleep disordered breathing?

Part of the concern is that breathing is supposed to occur through the nose, but when nasal congestion or blockages occur individuals start to breathe through their mouth. The mouth is the place where the dentist works, and when there are signs and symptoms of abnormal breathing in the mouth it is our duty to properly assess these and inform our patients. The other, more important factor, is that a person who breathes and sleeps better is generally much healthier. And that is the goal of Complete Health Dentistry, healthier whole people (not just mouths!).

We used to think bruxism (grinding of teeth) was caused primarily by psychological things (i.e. "stress"), but it is probably more of a mechanical release that helps people to not die of suffocation during sleep from their tongue being stuck back in the back of their throat.

When the jaw pushes forward it moves the tongue out of the way and they can breathe. Then as they fall asleep again the jaw and tongue will fall back again, and that is why they have a wearing down of the teeth as they scrape forward and backward against each other all night long in this constant teeth destructive yet life preserving cycle.

Another sign of a sleep breathing disorder that dentists can see is corrosion of the back teeth, commonly overlooked as simply "acid reflux". Stomach acid can become a vapor that comes up and into the back of the mouth. When the tongue gets stuck back in the throat during sleep it creates a negative pressure on the stomach and stomach acid, essentially pulling it up from the stomach and into the mouth the way a vacuum cleaner might. This can lead to a thinning of the teeth which is a corrosive or erosive wear on the teeth—meaning the teeth are actually dissolving.

So, if you don't sleep well, or you're tired during the day, you could be suffering from sleep disordered breathing. There are a wide range of symptoms and severity to sleep disordered breathing, including symptoms as seemingly small as having to wake multiple times during the night to use the restroom, and others listed below.

Adult Symptoms for Sleep-Disordered Breathing

- Headaches

- Snoring

- Difficulty sleeping

- Neck, jaw, or ear pain

- Sugar cravings

- Junk food cravings

- Obesity

- Type 2 diabetes

- Cardiovascular Disease

- Difficulty focusing mentally

- Excessive daytime sleepiness

- Low energy

- Wake up feeling unrefreshed

(Gelb and Hindin, <u>GASP</u>)

Cleansing Effects of Quality Sleep

"Ideal health, wellness, and brain development are dependent upon an open airway, nasal breathing, and deep, restorative sleep."

(Gelb and Hindin, <u>GASP</u>)

Scientists are discovering that the brain is constantly active until you're in deep non-REM sleep. The brain is astonishingly active during all of the other sleep phases. Dreaming sleep is important, but later in the sleep cycle is the non-REM rest where the brain itself gets to rest. This non-REM rest is vital for your brain's health, because this is when the brain gets the chance to shut down a little bit and get rid of all the debris that accumulate throughout the day.

The brain has neurotransmitters that make the brain work, allowing one cell to talk to another. Neurotransmitters are chemicals, and one cell makes and sends a neurotransmitter and another cell receives it. A few neurotransmitters you've probably heard of are norepinephrine, dopamine, serotonin, and many more, and they all have different functions. Once a neurotransmitter crosses the synapse (the gap between two cells) it has to be disposed of: either absorbed, broken down, or transported out of the pathway of the next neurotransmitter. If the used neurotransmitters aren't disposed of they clog up the pathway and you get misfires, or miscommunication from one cell to the next. The only time that this cleanup occurs is during sleep.

During deep non-**REM** sleep the blood brain barrier in the brain opens up to allow for self-cleansing. The brain's pathways get cleaned out of the debris that it built up during the day and now it can function without being sluggish. Sleep is the only thing that we know of that does that. A cup of coffee may make you feel bright temporarily, but it doesn't clean out the waste that is in there.

Deep sleep occurs early in the ninety minute sleep cycle if we are going to get deep sleep, and that is where the cleansing non-rem sleep occurs — as long as that part of the sleep cycle is completed. If that part of the cycle is interrupted and you awaken, the cleansing doesn't take place, and that is where you have what is called sleep fragmentation.

Symptoms of sleep fragmentation are so common that we make jokes about them. Frequently waking from sleep, frequent urination (yes this includes bed wetting), restless leg syndrome, sleep talking, and sleep walking can indicate sleep fragmentation. Believe it or not, your body might be trying to wake you up because it can't breathe.

And what happens when the non-**REM** sleep phase isn't completed? That neurotransmitter debris stays in there, and if it accumulates, it blocks communication from the brain to the body and vice versa. Like a scar that comes after an injury this debris remains in the way, and it is so common that it has a name: brain plaque.

And what do we call that blockage later on in life? We call it dementia, we call it Alzheimer's. Now synapses may be blocked, so instead of reacting properly to a situation, now we react aberrantly to it. Scientists are now asking: is it possible that good quality sleep can prevent these and other devastating diseases?

There are various psychological or neurological disorders modern medicine has tried to help with chemicals (medications), when there is a possibility that allowing that patient to rest may allow their body to repair itself. For the most part the brain can self-clean and regain health. There are very few diseases that occur in humans that the body can't clean up by itself.

Sleep Disordered Breathing has become a major focus of the dental industry because we work in the mouth every single day. Dentists can see signs that a larger issue may be occurring. It is our responsibility to inquire, educate, and direct our patients toward appropriate care. Since only physicians can order sleep tests, while dentists can not, then it is the dentist's responsibility to make you aware that a problem may exist and direct you to seek diagnosis and treatment that will positively affect your health. This again, is what complete health dentistry is all about.

At a checkup now, dentists are able to see signs or symptoms of a sleep breathing disorder, and we should bring this to the patient's attention. We should work in conjunction with the patient's primary physician to help this person rest better and breathe better. Dentists can and should positively affect not only the mouth but that patient's overall health.

There are a number of symptoms of sleep breathing disorders in kids too. Some symptoms that can indicate a breathing disorder are : crooked teeth, small mouths, arched palates, and thumb sucking. We need to assess if kids with these symptoms can breathe through their nose, or if they are forced to breathe through their mouths at all times.

Dentists can help people to use their nose for breathing, and yes, there are oral devices we can provide that can help with sleep breathing disorders.. There a lot of devices out there trying to help with sleep breathing disorders, but an oral device could be the best option for many people.

With all of this discussion about sleep you may be asking: what are optimal sleeping conditions?

In order to give yourself the best chance at high quality sleep (assuming you don't have a sleep disorder that needs additional treatment) try setting up your sleep station for success by making it: Cool. Dark. Quiet. Sleep specialists also recommend tv's and screens (phones, tablets) are turned off at least 90 minutes before going to sleep (this reduces stimulation by reducing bright light and noise specifically).

Diagnosing Sleep Disorders

"According to the National Institutes of Health, up to 70 million Americans are affected by chronic sleep disorders. Most People wouldn't think they're at risk, but what they don't realize is that anyone who hasn't had proper dental, jaw, or facial development is at risk."

(Dr. Steven Lin, <u>The Dental Diet</u>)

Sleep disorders are not just for drinking, smoking, overweight and middle-aged or older men.

All of those are factors than can contribute to the problem, but you aren't excluded if you aren't a part of those classifications. For example, look at Upper Airway Resistance Syndrome (UARS). In UARS breathing is not stopping, but there is resistance, and so you wake up, because your body thinks it is about to be suffocated from the airway resistance, and your fight or flight mode takes over and wakes you up. This is common in slender, fit people, particularly young women. They can be in bed for 8 hours, but never get good rest because they are falling asleep, getting resistance, and waking back up, rarely getting through a full 90 minute sleep cycle.

There are more than 80 known sleep disorders, but only a few have to do directly with breathing obstruction. Many symptoms that seem unrelated: chronic fatigue, fibromyalgia, and others that there is no "cure" for, seem to just go away or are significantly reduced when the patient begins to become well rested. If you can breathe, you can achieve restful sleep, if you can have restful sleep, you can become healthier.

There are two indices that are used to quantify and categorize sleep breathing disorders. The Apnea Hypopnea Index (AHI) is the main index used to designate the degree of obstructive sleep breathing. "Pnea" means breathing, "Apnea" means not breathing. Hypopnea means shallow breathing, which indicates some obstruction in the airway. Apnea is counted when the breathing stops for up to ten seconds, and it is measured as the number of times breathing stops per hour, not per night.

The second index is the Respiratory Distress Index (RDI). Like the AHI, the RDI collects data on Hypopnea and Apnea, but it also registers data on Respiratory Effort Related Arousals (RERA). RERA's include any occurrence that awakens you slightly, but without completely waking up.

There are multiple devices used to treat obstructed sleep breathing. The most common treatment is the use of a C-PAP machine. The C-PAP (which stands for Constant Positive Air Pressure) forces air into your nose and or mouth so that you get the oxygen you need. There are also many variations of oral devices that look similar to mouth guards. An Oral device stops your jaw from hanging back toward your throat and constricting the airway.

You might be surprised how much your jaw sliding back toward the throat can constrict your airway. To demonstrate just how far the jaw slides back, try this:

Close your eyes and close your mouth. Relax. Let your mouth open.

Tilt your head back and feel how your jaw slides back.

A properly fitted oral device will prevent your jaw from sliding back and closing the airway, allowing you to get better quality sleep.

Bacteria and Gum Disease

Inflammatory gum disease is the most common bacterial infection known to man, and those bacteria have immense ramifications on the vascular system throughout the body. We recognize that gum disease not only has an infection component, but also has an inflammation component, so the terms "gingivitis" and "periodontitis" are currently used to describe these conditions.

46% of American Adults Over 30 Show

Signs of Gum Disease

According to the Center for Disease Control (C.D.C.)

Symptoms of Periodontal Disease (or "Gum Disease")
From the American Dental Association (A.D.A.)

- Gums that bleed easily

- Red, swollen, tender gums

- Gums that have pulled away from the teeth (you may notice food getting stuck between the tooth and gum - as opposed to getting stuck in between teeth)

- Persistent bad breath or bad taste

- Permanent teeth that are loose or separating

- Any change to the way your teeth fit together when you bite

- Any change to the fit of partials or dentures

Gingivitis means "gums-inflammation".

Periodontitis means "tissues around the tooth — supporting bone, ligaments, and other connective tissues — inflammation".

But what predisposes a patient to these inflammatory conditions?

Why can one individual who never brushes, never flosses, or never eats correctly, have virtually no problems in the face of large amounts of bacteria?

And why can another individual who does everything possible to have a healthy mouth have major problems?

Let me be clear. Except for very few isolated circumstances, developing periodontal disease is your choice by ignoring your personal responsibilities to your overall health. There are, however, those certain circumstances where an infection begins in spite of your best intentions and actions.

In these circumstances it most often comes down to ecological balance of the patient's mouth and body. When the ecological balance is tipped one way or the other, that's when you get a susceptible host. And bang - you get disease.

But what if there is ecological balance?

For instance, I'm in contact every day with people who have illness to some degree or another. I rarely get sick, what's wrong (or right) with me? Am I not reacting? You've got to think of that as a possibility… or am I reacting in a way where I am so resistant that I don't acquire disease?

Nurses, physicians, those in the medical community rarely become sick. Why do we see that so often in the medical community? A major factor is that medical professionals often have good ecological balance, whereas someone who is ill is clearly out of ecological balance, but what does that mean? Let's look into that here using just the mouth as our window to understanding this concept.

The ecology of the oral cavity is created by combinations of the following factors:

- the amount, composition, consistency, and acidity of your saliva

- your dietetics

- your breathing habits

- your chewing, clenching and grinding habits

- your oral hygiene practices

- your drugs, medications, supplements regimens

- your smoking (any form or substance) or tobacco use tendencies

- your alcohol usage

- your tendency toward disordered sleep

- your age

- your personal fitness

Ecological balance has to do with the relationship between the microbial inhabitants of the oral cavity and the environment of the oral cavity. The mouth is known to harbor many hundreds of species of microbes including bacteria, protozoans, fungi, and viruses to name a few, with the population living in or on the oral tissues numbering in the millions. A microbe is anything that is a living organism that can be seen under a microscope or an electron microscope, meaning of course, that you can't see it in the mirror or with the naked eye.

When discussing common garden variety inflammatory gum disease, dentists are specifically dealing with a bacterial infection in the mouth. Different types of bacteria have different environemental requirements. There are three general types of bacteria that you need to understand, and even though there are thousands of bacterial strains, each strain will fall into one of these categories. There are *aerobes, facultative anaerobes,* and *obligatory anaerobes.*

You probably know that there are "good" bacteria and there are "bad" bacteria, but the third type are the truly "ugly" bacteria. Aerobes are usually the "good" bacteria. Aerobes prefer oxygen in their environment. The "bad" bacteria are facultative anaerobes. Facultative anaerobes can tolerate oxygen, but they prefer not to have it. And the worst bacteria, the "ugly", are obligatory anaerobes. Obligatory anaerobes can't tolerate any oxygen. In most situations anaerobic bacteria are more virulent in a negative way and cause more serious injury to the patient.

Now that we know what type of environment each type of bacteria prefers, we can intentionally change our mouth's ecology to help the "good" bacteria thrive, leaving little to no space for the "bad", or especially the "ugly" bacteria to live. But what if the "ugly" bacteria is already present? How do we change that environment, that ecology?

We can change that environment with some simple chemistry!

(Don't worry, I promise to keep it simple!)

A solution with 1.7% hydrogen peroxide is basically safe (6% or higher concentration will degrade anything it comes into contact with, and it is even more dangerous the higher percentage concentration it is). Hydrogen peroxide is a very unstable compound next to something that it can give up it's electrons to, meaning basically that it will give up it's oxygen. When it gives up oxygen electrons to another compound, it oxygenates that compound. Oxygenation of obligatory anaerobes (i.e. certain destructive "bad" bacteria) kills them.

It is possible to create an environment that is inhospitable to bad bacteria and simultaneously welcoming to good bacteria and lower your health risks. It is also possible for you to get oxygen into your system without any hydrogen peroxide, and reap those health benefits as well... and it has a lot to do with diet!

Human Ecology Basics

In high school biology, a small amount of time is spent on the topic known as ecology. Most students study this subject to pass a test, but few realize the real life ramifications of this topic when it comes to optimal health. It is estimated that the adult human body is composed of more than 10 trillion cells, but is inhabited by more than 100 trillion microbiotic organisms including bacteria, yeasts, and other single celled creatures. The basic relationship of ecology is a host (you and me, i.e. human species), an agent (our microbes), and suitable environmental factors (water, nutrients, and acid-base balance). When the ecology of our mouth is in appropriate balance, we consider our microbial partners to be beneficial. When the ecology of our mouth is out of balance, we consider our microbial partners to be pathogens, capable of producing disease reactions by us as the host.

Factors that Shift our Ecology from Health to Disease

This involves our heredity and the genes that make up our specific genetic expression. About 10% of our DNA is devoted to coding-specific proteins that either serve as anatomical building blocks or serve as enzymes that regulate our metabolism and growth/repair biochemical reactions. The other 90% of our DNA serves to code for proteins that either turn on or turn off genes, that allow for appropriate or disproportionate expression of regulatory genes.

The second factor is the relative composition of our resident microbial species. When beneficial species of microbes successfully compete for nutrients and places to live on their human host cells (and outnumber potentially harmful microbes), health exists. However, when conditions change in the oral environment the composition of our resident biome shifts to favor opportunistic species and then to pathogenic species, resulting in disease and dysfunction.

Some factors that can cause change in the oral environment are:

- increased sugar consumption,

- increased dry mouth (from medication or age-related decrease of saliva gland function),

- use of alcohol containing mouthwashes,

- use of broad spectrum antibiotics (from a prescription to combat infection, or consumed through antibiotic treated meats and poultry),

- lack of appropriate daily oral hygiene (brushing and flossing or water-flossing)

The third factor involves our own dietetics. It is estimated that the average adult American consumes more than 100 pounds of sugar annually. Some of this consumption is the result of using granulated sugar to sweeten everything from our morning coffee to our favorite desserts. But much of our sugar consumption comes under pseudonyms like dextrose, high fructose corn syrup, cane sugar, agave, and honey to name a few. When we increase the amount of sugar we consume, this tends to shift our resident microbes from mostly beneficial to increasingly detrimental. Additionally, the amount of water equivalent that we consume daily modifies our acid-base chemistry which regulates all of our host biochemical reactions.

Functional Medicine and
Functional Nutrition

"How should we deal with the growing problem
with our unhealthy food supply?...
Eat only natural anti-inflammatory foods. Support our
local farmers at the Farmer's Market."

(David R. Seaman, DC, MS, <u>The DeFlame Diet</u>)

The body is an ecology project, and the goal is to achieve and maintain balance, and thus achieve and maintain health. Homeostasis is the balancing act, and once in balance you stay in balance. If given a little too much sugar, the bad microbes (bacteria) that like sugar are going to grow a lot, and the good microbes that don't like sugar will get crowded out, creating imbalance. And when there are fewer of the good microbes then we can't get the vitamins they produce for us, making us more susceptible to decay or disease.

Two people can have a different rate of decay because patient "A" has a different type and amount of bacteria than the patient "B", and also because patient "B's" ecology is out of balance.

So how do we correct the balance, and bring the good microbes numbers back?

There are three common methods for changing the body's ecology: antibiotics, probiotics, and prebiotics.

When there is an infection that is overwhelming the body's own natural anti-infective inflammatory process we need to aid it, and we do that frequently with antibiotics. Antibiotics start to become ineffective because bacteria are so smart they become resistant to a specific antibiotic.

Bacterial genetic turnover (via reproduction) is occurring every twenty minutes or so, so you can have nearly a hundred generations in a 24 hour period. This means you can very rapidly have millions of bacteria that started out from just two. With each new generation of bacteria (just twenty minutes apart) comes a new slightly modified genetic code which allows them to become resistant to medications over generations.

This is why there have been (and will be) new antibiotics developed over time. It's important to understand that an antibiotic is not selective, it doesn't just go after bad bugs, it kills anything it can kill, including the collateral damage of good bugs. Unfortunately the good microbes and the bad microbes are going to die and it takes time for the good guys to grow back. This is why people sometimes get sick after an antibiotic, because the body's ecology is out of balance and the bad guys grow faster than the good guys.

So now you have a decimated microbial landscape of the internal of the gut as well as the rest of the body and you have to repopulate it. How? That's where probiotics and prebiotics come in. Probiotics are used to help the "good" bacteria repopulate before "bad" or "ugly" bacteria can get back into your system. Probiotics are commonly recommended for use when a patient needs to use an antibiotic, and can be found in yogurt, some fermented foods, or in a capsule or powder supplement form. Prebiotics are what the bacteria needs to live on. (I talked about the importance of getting fiber in our diet earlier in this book!) If we can proliferate the good bugs, you can get back into normal healthy tone again. It can take weeks to months or years to re-establish the healthy balance of bacteria that are in the gut, but we can assist them with probiotics and prebiotics.

Preserving a Healthy Ecology

"We cannot live without gut bacteria. In fact, there are actually far more bacteria in our gut than there are human cells that make up our bodies."

(David R. Seaman, DC, MS, <u>The DeFlame Diet</u>)

Many different probiotics are available in pharmacies and health food stores. The best contain no gluten or soy, are refrigerated, contain four or more different strains of beneficial bacteria, and report more than 1 billion live bacteria (cfu's) at the time of use. However, probiotic bacteria need nutrients and attachment sites, which bring the need for prebiotics. These are foods and preparations that support your healthy bacterial species and that contain high levels of fiber such as bran, fruits and vegetables.

Food Sources of Probiotics

- Yogurt

- Cabbage as sauerkraut, kimchi, or kapusta

- Miso soup

- Fremented soft cheeses (particularly Gouda, but also Swiss, cheddar and Parmesan)

It is important to note these foods do not cure illness by themselves. In conjunction with an anti-inflammatory diet, better health can be achieved. (David R. Seaman, DC, MS, <u>The DeFlame Diet</u>)

Alternative natural sweeteners give us a natural way to get the sweetness we crave in our foods without the bacterial growth promoting capabilities of sucrose (sugar) or its excess calories. Some examples of alternative natural sweeteners include erythritol, mannitol, and the five carbon sugar alcohol derived from the birch tree called xylitol. Xylitol is 6 times sweeter than sugar, comes in multiple forms (granulated, powdered), is bacteria-static (i.e. inhibits bacterial growth), and can be used by diabetics and prediabetics to help regulate blood sugar.

Vitamin K2

Around 80 years ago "vitamin K" was discovered to be involved in the clotting process. More recently, scientists realized that there were several different parts of the vitamin K molecule that looked similar but had different functions. Now renamed, vitamin K1 is involved with the clotting process. Vitamin K2, which we get from grass fed beef (Vitamin K2 comes from the chlorophyll in the grass the cows eat), or fremented foods like sauerkraut, is involved in calcium metabolism. (Vitamin K2 can also be created by bacteria in a lab, thus is also conveniently available in vitamin supplement form.)

Recently, to my complete shock, the husband of one of my long time hygienists relayed a conversation he had with his physician. He advised his doctor that he was taking vitamin K2 in supplement form. Not only had his doctor not heard of K2, but the patient now became the teacher, explaining the benefits of this vital nutrient to his primary care physician! Kudos to him! (And kudos to you for seeking out as much information as you can to impact your overall health!)

After World War II we started raising cattle on feed lots rather than making them eat grass, eliminating the chlorophyll from the cow's diet and consequently preventing us from getting vitamin K2 in the beef we consume. It was at this time that we began to see the increase and eventual spike of atherosclerosis, osteoporosis, diabetes, and cancer rates among American men and women. It is not a coincidence.

When we have a sufficient amount of vitamin K2 in our system the benefits of this protein modulator are many, including:

- Helps to regulate blood sugar levels that are so important in preventing diabetes

- Regulation of testosterone production

- Preventing atherosclerosis

- Preventing certain types of cancer

(From the book <u>Vitamin K2 and the Calcium Paradox</u>, Dr. Kate Rheaume-Bleue, BSc, ND)

It turns out vitamin K2 directs two proteins (Osteoclacin and Matrix GLA Protein), and they make sure the calcium goes where it is supposed to — into our bones and teeth, and not into our arteries. So vitamin K2 has a huge role in preventing atherosclerosis, the hardening of arteries — which is a major cause of heart attack. If you don't have the calcium deposits into the linings of the heart's arteries, they are going to function normally, allowing blood to flow with ease.

Vitamin K2 also has a huge role in preventing menopausal and post-menopausal women from becoming ostopenic and having osteomalacia. Diet again comes into play here, as women who are suffering any form of osteoporosis might have a vitamin K2 deficiency due to the lack of grass fed beef and or fremented foods in their diets. Calcium and vitamin D together are not enough.

Vitamin K2 may have positive effects in prevention of Alzheimer's disease too, because we know Alzheimer's disease also has a vascular component. If we can prevent the blood vessels in the brain from hardening through calcium deposits, we may have better blood flow and the buildup of the amyloid that forms in Alzheimer's disease may not form. Alzheimer's research is ongoing in this area.

How Complete Health Dentists Perform Check-Ups... And Why

"Doctors cannot give you health. Doctors can only remove symptoms or causes of symptoms; they cannot make you healthy! Becoming healthy is the job of the individual."

(David R. Seaman, DC, MS, <u>The DeFlame Diet</u>)

I believe in using the best possible diagnostics, so that I can determine the best possible course of treatment for each individual patient. I think about it in the same way a Chinese physician, about 4600 years ago did. He stated:

"The superior doctor prevents the disease.

The average doctor treats the disease in early stages.

The inferior doctor treats the disease when it is full blown."

I want to be a superior doctor for my patients. I want to prevent it before it's there.

One, it's less expensive. Two, it's less body invasive. And three, it's going to promote better overall health, and in the simplest possible way. It's a win-win-win situation!

Most people see their dental practitioners more than they see their regular physicians. Especially the male half of the population. Many adult males will only go to their primary care physician when something hurts, while almost everyone in our society will go the dentist at least twice a year for a "cleaning" and getting a check up. So dentists have a better chance to see signs and symptoms of what's going on at a check up, and can intercept a potential health risk at a much earlier time frame than a primary care physician might be able to. A sign is defined as when the practitioner recognizes that something isn't the way it ought to be, something is abnormal, rather than a variation of normal. A symptom is a patient report that something is wrong. Obviously a dentist isn't authorized to treat maladies that occur outside of their perview, but he or she can assess that a sign is present and refer a patient to a physician for an evaluation. That means dentists, as co-contributors with physicians, can help your overall health.

That leads dentists to investigate all kind of things in a patient's life, such as:

- whats going on in the stomach

- any breathing issues

- what toxic things are you doing to your mouth (like tobacco, alcohol, etc.)

- your working environment (working with abrasives or chemicals)

- having gum disease

- having teeth related problems

- amount of dietary sugar

Much of this information is gathered via conversation with the patient or through the use of surveys, like a medical history form, for example. Other information is gathered through visual and palpating inspection, the use of x-rays and high resolution photographs, and other quantitative measurements.

One thing we look at inside the mouth is the amount of saliva. You may not know this, but it is possible to have too much, or too little saliva in the mouth. As an example, in the winter, you can get dried out from being inside all the time. The dry climate causes sinus congestion, and instead of breathing through your nose, you're now breathing through the mouth — causing other ramifications (We discussed the benefits of breathing through the nose beginning on page 22 of this book!). On a different note, bacteria like to stick onto dry surfaces, so if there is no saliva, the bacteria take foothold and begin to proliferate, potentially sending your ecology out of balance and making illness possible, if not probable.

Keeping with the concept of Complete Health Dentistry, there are diagnostics dentists can perform (and we do routinely at your regular check up) that don't happen in the mouth that can signal health issues on your horizon.

We physically inspect by palpating the face, head and neck to see if there are areas that have muscle tension, have lymph node swelling, or other things like lesions, swellings, changes in chapped lips, or changes in moles and marks on the face and skin.

We will take your body temperature by running a temporal thermometer across your forehead. A high temperature is an immediate sign that there may be infection somewhere in your body, and possibly in the mouth.

We routinely do blood pressure analysis. Blood pressure is a sign that something is going on in the circulatory system. There are two numbers that we look at the systolic, the top number, which is the pressure thats generated when the heart contracts (pressure on). And diastolic, the bottom number, which is the pressure that is still in the blood vessels when the heart relaxes (pressure off). If the diastolic blood pressure is high that means the body isn't thoroughly relaxing. If the systolic blood pressure is high, it usually means the elasticity of the blood vessels has been diminished for some reason (calcification for example).

One Check-Up, Two Lives Saved!

A blood pressure reading is something we offer to all of our adult patients because signs of heart distress are not always visible to the naked eye.

We had a young woman come in for her check-up during her eighth month of pregnancy. Thankfully she consented to a blood pressure check, because her blood pressure was unusually high. I directed her to her physician right then and there. Her physician checked her blood pressure and immediately put her into the hospital — *she was that critical!*

Fortunately, she delivered and both she and the baby are fine. We saved two lives that day. And it was something as simple as checking her blood pressure.

We use a pulse oximeter, checking to see how well your blood is oxygenated. It should be over 96% oxygenation. Get below that and you get symptoms of oxygen deprivation. And we know that if the tissue doesn't get enough oxygen that tissue will die, leading to other serious health issues. We know smokers and those with other vascular disorders such as diabetes tend to have lower oxygenation. With diabetics, for example, if we don't protect the limbs early enough, then amputation becomes a real possibility. So using a pulse oximeter is a simple, painless test that indicates how much oxygen is getting to a peripheral tissue. If the blood oxygenation falls below 96% the heart has to beat faster and harder to try and get what little oxygen is there to the tissues that need it.

The pulse oximeter also checks how fast the heart is beating, and it should usually be 60-90 beats per minute. Tachycardia means "speeding heart" and means the heart rate is over 90 beats per minute. And if its lower than 60 beats per minute it is called bradycardia (pronounced "bratty cardia") or "slow heart". Those are both symptoms that alert us that something bad is, or will, occur.

At a checkup we will also observe your respiratory rate. A normal adult breathes between 12-20 times per minutes during a resting state. Fewer than twelve, or more than 20 breaths per minutes can indicate trouble with your heart and/or lungs.

One example of a health issue we are seeing more of is something called Metabolic Syndrome (sometimes referred to as Syndrome X, dysmetabolic syndrome, or insulin resistance syndrome). We see signs at a much earlier stage than the physicians do because we are seeing you so regularly. We develop that relationship — especially our hygienists, because they get to spend an hour at each visit with you, they get to know you, and can see changes in your health. Plus, our routine diagnostics that seem to have little to do with dentistry allow us to see signs of problem areas in your health.

What is Metabolic Syndrome?

Metabloic Syndrome is a combination of factors that increase your risk of heart attack, stroke, and diabetes. Factors include: being overweight, having high blood pressure, abnormal heart rate and respiratory rate, bad blood sugar and a1c levels, and increased waist circumference.

Cutting Edge Diagnostics

While it is not difficult for a dentist to diagnose inflammatory gum disease, finding and eliminating the root cause is not always easy. We have had patients with inflammatory gum disease whom we could not figure out. Their mouths didn't have a heck of a lot of plaque. But every time they were in, we would touch the gums and they would bleed. And these are pretty healthy individuals otherwise, but the gums would bleed which tells us something's not right.

For years dentists would refer them to the periodontist who would say "Let's scrape them better, and teach them to be better at home hygiene." And yes, removing the plaque and tartar that the harmful bacteria lived in was probably helpful, but it wasn't solving the problem. It was only disrupting the symptoms. Visit after visit we would keep seeing the same results even with better, and more frequent, traditional care. We needed to take a look from a different point of view.

During my search for a better result I read as many books and articles as I could find, and on many weekends I would travel to hear speakers at clinics whom I thought could help me find the answer I was looking for. I met Tobias Hain at a "No More Hygiene" presentation in 2017. Tobias Hain is the founder of Hain Diagnostics in Germany. He developed a way of testing to discover what kind of bacteria live in your mouth that are causing your particular gum disease. This is invaluable, because there are over

700 types of bacteria found in human mouths, and some bacterial mixtures are very, very destructive.

"The Good, The Bad, and The Ugly... Bugs"

When categorizing bacteria Hain Diagnostics differentiates bacteria into colored groups: red, orange, yellow, and green. With more than 700 species of bacteria in our mouths at all times, we use the color code as a way to quickly decipher the level of danger the particular group of species presents to a specific host patient. As a general rule, if there isn't enough oxygen in the environment of the bacteria, then you're going to get the worse bugs; if more oxygen you're going to get the better bugs.

The orange, yellow, and green grouped bugs are less pathogenic by themselves, meaning they are not tissue destructive without help. The green group is comprised of "good bugs", and can actually assist us in a symbiotic relationship. The yellow and orange groups are made up of "bad bugs". The orange group "bad bugs" are bacteria that when they associate with "ugly bugs" in the red group, they become more dangerous. By themselves they're bad, but when they associate with "ugly bugs" they're very bad. If we start to see a little gum puffiness we know something is going on... but we don't necessarily know which bacteria are present and causing the issue.

The red group includes just one type of bacteria — Aggregatibacter actinomycetemcomitans ("Aa", for short), the "ugly bug". This bacteria, "Aa", all by itself invades body tissue and starts to cause the body to want to degrade itself to get away from the bacteria. Being tissue invasive does not mean that it will get directly inside the teeth, but it will get inside the gums and the attachment mechanism for the teeth, and into the bone. It is difficult to get inside the tooth, it would have to get in by the blood supply.

Now, what's interesting about it is, if "Aa" is present you will have bleeding gums and start to get bone destruction — *even if you don't have a lot of plaque.* "Aa" is only found in the mouth as an infection, however the infection isn't like when you have an infection on your hand where you can see it. In the mouth it's hidden, and the only time you'd find it yourself is when you're brushing and you've got bleeding. But that bleeding is a late stage effect, meaning the infection has been present in your mouth for some time.

Up until now the only thing we could do to combat these bugs was to do scrapings, and clean the gums off, clean the bacteria-laden stuff off, and hope like heck that your body takes over. Now, due to this cutting edge bacterial DNA test we can differentiate between the bacteria that are present and devise a plan to deal with each patient's own cocktail of bacteria.

With the information gained from this diagnostic test, we can prescribe an antibiotic that will kill the bacteria and then, hopefully the rest of the bacterial spectrum will change for the better. A healthier bacterial spectrum and you'll get healthier, not only in the gums, but also in the bones that hold your teeth and also throughout your body.

We had one patient that continued to have bleeding at each visit, no matter what care was provided by us or the periodontist. So Deb, our lead hygienist, had this patient in, and did the test. The results were life changing! He had "Aa", the worst bug of all, and a large amount — which you could not tell by looking at him.

Once we knew the cause of his gum disease, we could say, "Here is what we can do for you if you are willing to try and stop this disease. Not only can we stop it in your mouth, but we're probably going to improve the whole rest of your body as well."

We know we can help him live a healthier life, because we know that "Aa" is linked to at least 50% of the cases of sudden cardiac arrest. "Aa" has been found in atheromas — the blood clots that form within the heart that cause atherosclerosis which lead to heart attacks.

And he's a pretty healthy guy already, to start with, late 40's, we've been working on his gum disease treatment for a long time and tried all kinds of different ways to see if we can correct it, without knowing that the "ugly bug" was the culprit. We had tried dietetics issues, we thought maybe he was low in vitamin C, sometimes we'll see capillary bleeding, it helped, but wasn't the whole solution. Knowing the root cause of his issues was a game changer — and there is no other way to know that than by performing a bacterial DNA test. We know that if we get rid of the bacteria that's causing the problem, then the disease goes away. No "bad bugs", no "ugly bugs", no disease.

The bacterial testing process is simple and painless. What you do is you take a sample of the bacteria that are in a person's mouth on a sterile paper point. Take five of these little paper points and just touch the gums where the bacteria are and then seal the paper point into a test tube that gets shipped to the Hain Diagnostics testing center.

Within ten days we get a full report on what's in your mouth that reveals the type and relative amounts of these bacteria. The report will show if the bacteria are above the tissue destructive threshold, or if the bacteria is relatively safe and non-threatening. This allows us to distinguish what's going on with precise diagnostics so that we can treat the specific cause of the infection rather than treating just the symptoms the infection created. It also allows us to customize treatment to each individual patient.

Bacterial DNA testing is relatively inexpensive. It is only a matter of time before most insurances will cover it. My suspicion is that once it becomes a commonly offered diagnostic test, they probably will cover it, especially because it is relatively inexpensive when compared to costly late stage disease treatment.

Unfortunately, at this time you probably can't walk into any dentist and ask for this testing. They're probably not set up to offer it. They may not have that connection with the diagnostics companies.

We have opted to do that. Our team is ready and rearing to go, to offer this test as part of our care to help not only the mouth, but the whole body. We understand we can help people live longer, healthier lives.

Gum Disease and Complete Health Connection

"Nearly 75 million Americans have unhealthy gums, which can nearly double the risk of a heart attack... and many of them don't realize it, because an oral infection is painless in the early stages."

(Bale and Doneen, Beat the Heart Attack Gene)

It is so important that dental practitioners remember to educate patients on how dangerous gum disease truly is to their health.

If you brushed your hair and started to bleed from the scalp you'd know something was wrong. If you scratched your hand you'd put anti-bacterial stuff on the scratch.

But if you brush your teeth and have bleeding, all you do is spit it out and say, "It's only a little bleeding." That's crazy.

That blood you spit out tells me that something is wrong, and your body is trying to fight it. If blood is getting out, then that means bacteria can get in. If bacteria can get into the blood, then these bacteria are going to the heart. It's going to the liver. It's going to the brain. It's going to every single organ.

Up to 50% of sudden death from cardiac arrest is attributable to the bacteria in the mouth. The same bacteria causing that person's gum disease has traveled through the blood system to the heart, because the whole body is connected by the vascular system, the blood vessels.

Two prominent individuals in this field are Dr. Brad Bale and Dr. Amy Doneen, the co-authors of a book called <u>Beat the Heart Attack Gene</u> (I highly recommend this book if you have a family history of heart disease — it talks about many more factors for heart attack than periodontal disease). They also authored the definitive paper on the connection of the bacteria of the mouth and heart disease in 2016. Their study absolutely linked the bacteria from periodontitis with atherosclerosis in the heart. Atherosclerosis is the hardening of the arteries, a closing of the arteries that leads to myocardial infarction (heart attack). Periodontal disease used to be an "associated" risk for a heart attack. Now periodontal disease is recognized as a one to one causal relationship. In other words, *the bacteria in the mouth causes this problem in the heart*. It is not a coincidence any more. It is a definite link.

There are more connections between the infection in the mouth we call periodontal disease or inflammatory gum disease and the diseases found throughout the body. We already connected the dots to heart disease above, but there are links to each of the following diseases as well: lung disease, brain disease, there's implication on Alzheimer's here, pancreatic disease, and certain cancers of the digestive track.

And people that are at high risk for these diseases, including inflammatory gum disease, are people who have vascular disease already. Diabetes is a vascular disease. This is why so many people lose limbs or go blind, because once you don't get oxygenation, the tissue dies. It's an intimate connection.

There is another oral bacteria that has been implicated in low birth weight babies and still born births, because it can transfer from the parent through the placenta to the fetus — yet another vascular connection.

It seems to me, with the mouth being a window into the rest of the body, that going to a Complete Health Dentist and having the proper diagnostic evaluations done would be the least invasive way to find out what some of those risks are... I know I'd prefer to find out what's going on inside my body without needles, exploratory surgeries, or biopsies.

Diagnosing Periodontal Disease

Periodontal disease is sneaky — silently invading your mouth and taking root before causing massive destruction. Periodontal disease has no symptoms at the beginning stages, therefore many people are unaware they have it. There are signs of later stage periodontal disease you can recognize for yourself (See page 39 for a list), but your best bet for early detection is to make sure you don't miss or delay your regular dental check-ups.

Even though dental diagnostic methods are primitive, they are effective. At this point in human history the best we can offer in terms of diagnostics is using our measurement tool, and checking for bleeding. X-rays are useful tools, unfortunately bone loss only shows up on the x-ray when the change from the background to change is more than 30% — so you can have 30% disease attrition and it doesn't show up on an x-ray yet. Think about that — nearly one-third of the bone has been destroyed and x-rays cannot confirm it. (Imagine if you didn't believe your dentist's diagnosis and waited another six months for x-ray "proof"... how much damage could be done by then?)

Dentists are trying to treat the patient before they have bone loss. Imagine dentists' frustration with insurance companies who want x-ray "proof" of bone loss before approving coverage of periodontal disease treatment, when bone destruction is less than that thirty percent threshold that is visible on an x-ray. (Not to mention that it is going to cost everyone less money in the long run because healthier patients cost less to care for than sick patients.)

Even without the visual "proof" of periodontal disease x-rays provide in later stages, dentists use other methods of diagnosis to verify its presence, crude as they may be. Dentists look for a measured loss of bone tissue over time by checking current measurements against your older (or even original) measurements and seeing the amount of bone loss that has occurred. We also look for bleeding along the measurement sites and general swelling (among other signs). (Are there people who bleed without periodontal disease? Yes, but it's because something else is going on, which is rare.) At times we will even perform a bacterial DNA test to determine what bacteria are present in your mouth.

Treating periodontal disease and reducing inflammation in the gums will help reduce inflammation in the blood vessels and throughout the body.

In case you were wondering, there is a common diagnostic test that every dental office should be using in care of their patients. Your hygienist should be measuring your gum health at least once each year. This is a simple process where a rubber-tipped probe is placed next to each tooth to measure how snug and tight your gums are holding your teeth.

If you are unsure about the probe, have the hygienist let you touch it to your fingertip (I promise it will not hurt!). Measuring your gums won't hurt you either... Unless there is a gum infection present (in which case it can be sensitive to the touch---and a great hygienist will minimize the pain for you as much as possible).

While moving from tooth to tooth your hygienist will be announcing measurements (in millimeters) and stating where they see bleeding, if there is any. It may sound like this: "...tooth number 24, 3 (millimeters), 2mm, 4mm, bleeding on medial...". <u>The whole process should take less than 2 minutes.</u>

Any measurements between 1mm and 3mm are considered normal and healthy. If those are your measurements Congratulations! Just remember, those numbers aren't static and can change in a matter of months, and the longer you go between check-ups with your hygienist the greater risk you have of infection.

If your measurements are 4mm or higher, you may need more advanced hygiene care, and need care more frequently.

Possibly the best way to find periodontal disease at the earliest possible moment is a blood test for High Specificity C Reactive Protein (HSCRP). HSCRP is a general inflammatory marker. This informs us that there is inflammation in your system, and where is inflammation most common? In the gum tissue in the mouth, in the digestive tract, or arthritis. If we can find inflammation earlier we can prevent it from becoming disabling — regardless of it's location in the body (mouth, gut, hands, etc.).

Disease and Tooth Loss

Aside from trauma, there are two primary diseases that cause tooth loss in adults. One, is Caries Disease (cavity disease), the other is Periodontal Disease (gum disease). Cavities and gum disease are the 2 most common diseases affecting human beings. If Caries Disease is untreated long enough there can eventually be enough damage that the tooth is both painful and unsaveable. If Caries Disease causes tooth removal, the removal of the tooth solves the issue and health can be regained after healing of the surgical site is complete.

If Periodontal Disease causes sufficient bone loss, the tooth will still need to be removed. The difference is, the disease that caused the damage may still be present and active after the tooth's removal, and even after a replacement is there (e.g.- an implant). The next logical question is can you lose an implant? Yes. If the periodontal disease is still active at that site it is called perio-implantitis, and will still cause damage to the bone around the implant, causing the implant to lose stability, and if untreated, the implant will have to be removed.

The Truth About Preventive Hygiene Visits

"You want us on that wall! You need us on that wall!"

(<u>A Few Good Men</u>, Aaron Sorkin)

The commonly accepted practice of having a "cleaning" twice a year isn't optimal for the overwhelming majority of people. To truly prevent disease people should be seen every 90 days, because bacteria can become harmful for someone who isn't doing a good job with home hygiene care (brushing and flossing). In 24 hours there is enough bacteria that they'll begin to make calculus (calcium hardened houses) and then they'll go to work on your teeth. The primary reason to go to a hygiene visit is education — to discover early on if there are problems. To learn what the problems are, mitigate those problems or learn how to prevent them. And yes, we do some "housekeeping" to remove calculus buildup.

Every extra month between visits can really add up exponentially in terms of damage (remember, a new generation of bacteria is produced about every twenty minutes) and financial costs. The American public spends billions of dollars in healthcare annually, and people need to understand that having healthy mouths would improve their general health. Just using a toothbrush and floss regularly would greatly reduce medical costs (more on brushing and flossing in a bit).

And so, with great wisdom, most people come into our office when they are healthy and looking to prevent future tooth, gum, and jaw breakdowns. That's the idea behind regular hygiene check ups and "cleaning" visits (the real term for that process is "prophylaxis", which means "action taken to prevent disease"). Professional "cleaning" is the only effective way to remove those rock-hard plaque deposits (calculus) from your teeth and evict the bacterial colonies that are housed there. Removing that bacterial buildup will allow you the opportunity to get your mouth's ecology back into balance.

At Home Care

*"A habit that takes five minutes a day... brushing and
flossing your teeth... can add years to your life and also
reduces risk for heart attacks, strokes, diabetes, colds, flu, and even arthritis."*

(Bale and Doneen, Beat the Heart Attack Gene)

How do we keep the mouth's ecology balanced in between dental hygiene visits?

Maintaining a healthy mouth ecology is primarily done through regular brushing and flossing after meals to remove excess loose bacteria and their food supply that is left behind after eating. When brushing use a toothbrush with rounded soft ends, and be sure the head of your toothbrush is only large enough to brush a maximum of two teeth at a time. If your bristles are too hard, or if you are scrubbing too hard, you can abrade the tissues of the teeth and the gums. Last, but not least, when you brush you should sweep, rather than scrape.

To get in between the teeth we can floss (or use dental tape if you prefer) to dislodge the colonization of bacteria that are on the tooth, and remaining food particles. The problem is that floss is a straight line device and teeth aren't straight lined, they're curved, so what happens is this, sometimes you hit some surfaces, and sometimes you hit others.

Waterpik irrigating spritz (or any water-flosser) can get in and dislodge food particles and new bacterial colonies, and get rid of the debris. Water irrigators also massage the gum tissue. Anybody who has ever had a massage knows how good that feels, and whats happening you're improving oxygenation and circulation by working the soft tissue.

Additional Recommendations for Maintaining a Healthy Ecology

Toothpaste **without surfactants** (surfactant is something that makes things slippery, so when they make debris slippery, the debris comes off, and the slippery feel helps it stay off. Too mush surfactant and it takes off some of the stuff you want to be there [i.e. good bacteria].)

Mouthwash **without alcohol** (alcohol kills good and bad bacteria, dries the mouth tissues and makes them sticky, so bacteria that wasn't supposed stick, sticks, and you've restarted a cycle of bad bacteria growth)

What About Fluoride?

Enamel is the hardest substance in the human body. If bacteria can destroy enamel, imagine what damage those same bacteria can do to the rest of the body once it's in your bloodstream, being pumped from organ to organ with each heartbeat.

Here's the big question on fluoride — How much is not good for you? Fluoride in large amounts is toxic. So is water (you can drown). The thing itself isn't the problem, it's the amount that can be excessive (think: sugar, alcohol, junk food).

The American Dental Association (ADA) advocates for the use of fluoride in toothpaste, drinking water, and in topical treatments on our teeth. In a chemical process, fluoride changes the structure of the tooth's enamel so that acids can't dissolve it as easily. Part of bacterial metabolism is the excretion of acid. Acid leaches calcium out of material that contains it, like enamel. This begins cavity formation, and then you don't have long before you have a hole in the tooth, or cavity.

To combat the assault of bacterial-waste (acid) we introduce fluoride to the equation.

While the enamel is forming, fluoride incorporates into the enamel — making it more resistant to bacterial degradation.

Enamel is primarily made from a material called calcium hydroxyapatite. When fluoride is involved some of the hydroxide radicals get substituted for the fluoride ion and incorporated into the now stronger enamel — and then the acid can't dissolve it as easily. It doesn't work as well on dentin (the next layer of the tooth inside the enamel) because there is less calcium hydroxyapatite in dentin to begin with, therefore fewer places for fluoride ions to be swapped in to.

If you ingest fluoride and it is incorporated into the building of the enamel the whole thickness of the enamel gets to have added strength. Fluoride also changes the shape of the surface of the tooth so that there are less grooves, meaning fewer places for bacteria to congregate. When you apply fluoride topically, only the surface of the enamel is strengthened. Once that surface is breached the cavity will begin to grow at a faster rate.

Think of it this way. If you were to pour a foundation for a house, and you put blue paint into the cement, the finished product will have blue paint incorporated into the entire thickness of the cement. This is similar to the result of ingesting fluoride through your drinking water, in that the entire thickness of the enamel will have fluoride within it. However, if you pour a foundation and then paint it blue, the paint is only on the surface of the cement. This is analogous to placing a topical fluoride treatment on your teeth. Having both treatments being done regularly offers the best chance for strong enamel protecting your teeth.

7 More Years!

"Just flossing alone would add seven years to your life."

(Mike Rouzine from the Cleveland Clinic)

Seven years is almost ten percent added on to an average American's life expectancy.

Ten percent! Imagine how much more time that gives you to enjoy your family and friends... And imagine you are healthy the whole time! What new experiences and adventures will you have?

What would it be worth to you to be healthier for an extra seven years?

To see your kids grow up? Graduate? Get married? Have children of their own? See your grandchildren graduate and get married?

Would it be worth it for you to learn about your health, and then spend 4 minutes a day applying what you learn?

There are 168 hours in a week for each of us... I don't want to hear that you don't have time to brush and floss. Make it a priority for yourself, for your loved ones.

And make an appointment for a hygiene check-up* today.

(*If you are long overdue it is especially important to find a dental team that won't make you feel judged. For more information about my office, go to www.SouthWindsorSmiles. com)

Yes, Cavities and gum disease are the two most common diseases affecting humans, but the inflammatory response these diseases trigger are not contained to the mouth. The inflammatory response is probably occurring elsewhere because the body has a standard operating procedure. If it is happening in the mouth it is happening somewhere else in the body. This makes the mouth a great window to the body because the mouth is easy to get access to — and your dentist should recognize these signs and educate you about your health.

It is *your health.* **Take charge!** Don't let someone else drive your vehicle. Prevention of disease is the most effective health care. Everything else is sick care. Make continuous efforts to practice health care — eat a healthy diet, get regular vigorous exercise, get quality rest, get regular check-ups with your primary care physician and dentist, and please take a few minutes every day to brush and floss — you won't regret it!

Dear Reader,

Hopefully, if you've made it this far, you've found this book interesting and easy to digest. There is a wealth of information available to help us understand what to do to obtain true health — and there is more information coming out all the time!

Let me be the lens that clarifies the astounding amount of information available to you about your health. If your organization has a specific area of concern, a tailored presentation can be created to suit your needs.

They say variety is the spice of life, and I've. Found that to be true. I have enjoyed speaking to varied audiences, from health professionals to laymen, from children to senior citizens.

Looking forward to discussing the connection of dentistry to overall health with you and your group. Until then, wishing you the best of health.

— Dr. Kevin H. Norige

For more information on booking Dr. Norige as a speaker, visit:
www.Kevin-Norige.com

Get a pretty cool bonus while you're there! Nope... No hints! You'll have to go check it our for yourself. You can thank me later.

*Offer subject to change without notice